# Candida Albicans

## A Beginner's 5-Step to Managing the Condition Through Diet and Other Home Remedies, With Sample Recipes

**mf**

# Disclaimer

By reading this disclaimer, you are accepting the terms of the disclaimer in full. If you disagree with this disclaimer, please do not read the guide.

All of the content within this guide is provided for informational and educational purposes only, and should not be accepted as independent medical or other professional advice. The author is not a doctor, physician, nurse, mental health provider, or registered nutritionist/dietician. Therefore, using and reading this guide does not establish any form of a physician-patient relationship.

Always consult with a physician or another qualified health provider with any issues or questions you might have regarding any sort of medical condition. Do not ever disregard any qualified professional medical advice or delay seeking that advice because of anything you have read in this guide. The information in this guide is not intended to be any sort of medical advice and should not be used in lieu of any medical advice by a licensed and qualified medical professional.

The information in this guide has been compiled from a variety of known sources. However, the author cannot attest to or guarantee the accuracy of each source and thus should not be held liable for any errors or omissions.

You acknowledge that the publisher of this guide will not be held liable for any loss or damage of any kind incurred as a result of this guide or the reliance on any information provided within this guide. You acknowledge and agree that you assume all risk and responsibility for any action you undertake in response to the information in this guide.

Using this guide does not guarantee any particular result (e.g., weight loss or a cure). By reading this guide, you acknowledge that there are no guarantees to any specific outcome or results you can expect.

All product names, diet plans, or names used in this guide are for identification purposes only and are the property of their respective owners. The use of these names does not imply endorsement. All other trademarks cited herein are the property of their respective owners.

Where applicable, this guide is not intended to be a substitute for the original work of this diet plan and is, at most, a supplement to the original work for this diet plan and never a direct substitute. This guide is a personal expression of the facts of that diet plan.

Where applicable, persons shown in the cover images are stock photography models and the publisher has obtained the rights to use the images through license agreements with third-party stock image companies.

# Table of Contents

# Introduction

Imagine waking up every day feeling exhausted and drained, unable to determine what's causing this discomfort. Here's one suggestion: Candida Albicans. If you experience recurring yeast infections, digestive issues, and skin irritations that seem to have no end, these are usually caused by Candida Albicans. This condition plagues countless women worldwide. About 75% of women in the United States experience Candida Albicans once in their lifetime at the very least.

Understanding Candida Albicans and its detrimental effects on your body is the first step toward finding long-lasting solutions. By delving into the causes, symptoms, and treatment options available, you can gain the upper hand in combating this stubborn condition.

No woman should have to endure the discomfort and frustration caused by Candida Albicans. By gaining comprehensive knowledge about this condition, you can take control of your health and make informed decisions.

Imagine living a life free from the debilitating symptoms of Candida Albicans, where energy and vitality become your new norm. This guide will equip you with the tools necessary to embark on a journey towards optimal health and well-being.

In this Guide, we will talk about the following:

- What Is Candida Albicans?
- Causes and Risk Factors of Candida Albicans
- Symptoms of Candida Albicans
- Home Remedies, Medical Treatments, and Lifestyle Changes to Manage Candida Albicans
- What Is Candida Albicans Diet?
- Principles, Benefits, and Disadvantages of Candida Albicans
- Step-Guide to Get Started with the Candida Albicans Diet
- Foods to Eat and To Avoid
- Sample Recipes and Meal Plan

Get ready to dive deep into the world of Candida Albicans. In the upcoming chapters, we will explore the causes and risk factors associated with this condition. We will unveil the telltale signs and symptoms that may be sabotaging your daily life. Keep reading to discover the various medical and home treatment options available, as well as how to manage this condition through diet.

# All About Candida Albicans

Candida Albicans is a yeast type of fungus that naturally occurs in the body. It lives on human skin, intestines, and other mucous membranes. Women typically have more of this bacteria than men because it thrives in warm and moist areas such as the vagina. Candida itself is yeast in the body regulated by the body's microbiome or good bacteria.

When Candida Albicans grows out of control, the result is an overgrowth of yeast in the body. This can lead to a wide range of uncomfortable and irritating symptoms.

Here is an important detail about Candida albicans. It is NOT a sexually transmitted infection. The Candida yeast naturally occurs in the body that reacts when there's lack of good bacteria to regulate it. While performing sexual activity may disturb the balance of the yeast in the body, it is not the lead cause of the infection.

## Symptoms

There are various ways to determine if you have Candida Albicans. While it's best to consult a health professional, it's also good to be aware of the symptoms of Candida Albicans. These may be observed in different parts of the body, not only around and inside the vagina and rectum but also including the insides of the mouth and throat, on the folds of the skin in the groin, arms, and under the breasts. As for infants and children, around the diaper region, such as the buttocks, genitals, and thighs.

## Vaginal itching or soreness

This yeast overgrowth disrupts the vaginal pH balance and irritates. Other symptoms may include a thick, white discharge, burning during urination, and pain during sex.

Treatment options include antifungal medications, probiotics, and dietary changes. It is important to seek medical advice if symptoms persist or worsen.

## Pain during sexual intercourse

You may experience swelling, redness, itching, and burning in the vaginal area, making penetrative sex uncomfortable and even painful. In addition to physical discomfort, this symptom can also lead to emotional distress and strain on intimate relationships.

## Pain or discomfort when urinating

This infection can also trigger itching and burning sensations around the genitals, as well as cause white, thick discharge. It is important to seek medical attention if these symptoms persist or worsen.

## Abnormal vaginal discharge

The discharge is usually thick, and white, and resembles cottage cheese. It can also be accompanied by burning, itching, and soreness in the genital area. It's important to seek medical attention for proper diagnosis and treatment.

## Skin redness (rash)

Notice redness in the moisture-prone areas of your body like the groin and under your breasts. This type of skin rash is caused by the overgrowth of the yeast and can result in itching and discomfort.

## Lumpy white patches

Also known as oral thrush, this condition manifests as lumpy white patches on the tongue or inside of the mouth. Those with weakened immune systems, diabetes, or those taking antibiotics are more susceptible to oral thrush.

It's important to note that these symptoms can also be indicative of other conditions, so it's best to consult a healthcare professional for an accurate diagnosis and appropriate treatment.

# Causes and Risk Factors

There are various factors that cause Candida Albicans, and here are some common causes:

## Imbalanced Vaginal Flora

Also known as vaginal dysbiosis. The vaginal environment is primarily composed of healthy bacteria known as lactobacilli, which maintain the vaginal pH level in a slightly acidic range. This acidic environment helps to prevent the overgrowth of harmful bacteria and yeast.

## Weakened Immune System

Certain conditions or medications can interfere with the body's ability to fight off infections, including the overgrowth of yeast. Women with autoimmune disorders, such as HIV or lupus, are more prone to Candida infections.

## Hormonal Changes

Increased levels of estrogen, progesterone, and other hormones during pregnancy, menopause, or the menstrual cycle can create an environment that supports Candida growth.

## Antibiotics

When someone takes antibiotics, it can have a major impact on the natural bacterial balance within the body. This changes the pH level and makes it easier for the growth of Candida

Albicans, a fungus that is typically harmless in small amounts. Women are more susceptible to this fungal infection than men because of the natural pH level of the vagina.

## High Sugar Intake

When sugar and refined carbohydrates are consumed in excess, they serve as a source of fuel for Candida, encouraging its multiplication and leading to an increased risk of infection.

Furthermore, Candida thrives in a high-acidic environment, and the metabolization of sugar creates an acidic environment, providing an optimal environment for Candida's growth.

## Tight or Damp Clothing

This happens because such clothing creates a warm and moist environment that encourages the growth of Candida.

Additionally, wearing tight clothing also reduces the amount of air that circulates to the genitals, which can worsen any existing yeast infection symptoms.

## Uncontrolled Diabetes

Additionally, uncontrolled diabetes can lead to decreased immune function and impaired wound healing, which can also contribute to an increased risk of Candida albicans infections in women.

Women with diabetes should therefore ensure that they keep their blood sugar levels well-controlled to reduce the risk of developing candidiasis. Proper diabetes management can not only help prevent Candida infections but also improve overall health outcomes.

It's important to note that while these factors can contribute to Candida Albicans in women, individual experiences may vary. It is advisable to consult with a healthcare professional for an accurate diagnosis and appropriate treatment.

# Women and the Infection

As opposed to popular knowledge, Candida Albicans affect women of all ages, not just adults. The different symptoms and risk factors mentioned in the previous chapter may manifest on different ages of women. Below are some of these symptoms that manifest on different ages:

**Vaginal yeast infection**

Mainly common on adult women, particularly those who take hormones pills or birth control pills. Those who are pregnant also experience this infection, as well as those who have weak immune system or had to take antibiotics.

**Oral thrush**

Infants, children, and older adults may have this. Those who have compromised immune system, as well as those who wear dentures.

**Invasive candidiasis**

Patients who end up having this usually are those who are hospitalized for various medical reasons, surgery patients, with compromised immune system, as well as those who use catheters.

# Medical Treatment for Candida Albicans

There are several medical treatments available to address Candida Albicans infections, including;

- **Antifungal medications**: The primary treatment for Candida Albicans infections involves the use of antifungal medicines. These medications work by targeting and eliminating the fungal infection to prevent further overgrowth. They can be prescribed in the form of topical creams, ointments, sprays, or oral fluconazole for systemic infections.

- **Azoles**: Azoles are a class of antifungal agents commonly used to treat Candida Albicans infections. They are preferred and frequently prescribed due to their effectiveness in combating the fungus. Depending on the severity and type of infection, different azole drugs such as fluconazole, miconazole, or clotrimazole may be used.

- **IV antifungal therapy**: In cases of severe or invasive Candida Albicans infections, intravenous (IV) administration of antifungal medications like fluconazole, caspofungin, or micafungin may be necessary. IV therapy allows for direct delivery of the medication into the bloodstream to combat widespread or systemic infections.

- **Rezafungin**: Recently approved by the FDA, rezafungin is a new treatment option for invasive candidiasis. It has shown promise in clinical trials and offers an alternative for patients who may not respond to traditional antifungal therapies. Rezafungin is administered through injection.

- **Candida cleanse diet**: While not a medical treatment per se, some individuals may opt for the candida cleanse diet as an adjunct to their treatment plan. This diet involves avoiding certain foods that promote yeast growth, such as sugar and refined carbohydrates, and focusing on a balanced, nutrient-rich meal plan to support overall health and immune function.

It is important to consult with a healthcare professional for an accurate diagnosis and appropriate treatment plan tailored to individual needs.

# Managing Candida Albicans

To manage Candida Albicans in women, making certain lifestyle changes can be beneficial. Here are some lifestyle changes that may help:

- **Maintain proper hygiene**: Keeping the vaginal area clean with mild, unscented soap and water can help prevent Candida overgrowth.
- **Follow a Candida diet**: The Candida diet involves eliminating foods that may promote the growth of Candida yeast, such as sugar, gluten, alcohol, and certain dairy products. This can help create an environment less conducive to Candida overgrowth.
- **Avoid tight-fitting clothing**: Wearing loose-fitting clothing allows for better airflow and can help prevent moisture buildup, which can contribute to Candida growth.
- **Change out of wet clothing promptly**: Moist environments provide an ideal breeding ground for Candida. Changing out of wet clothing, such as swimwear or sweaty gym clothes, can help reduce the risk of infection.

- **Manage stress levels**: High levels of stress can weaken the immune system, making women more susceptible to Candida overgrowth. Implementing stress management techniques, such as exercise, meditation, or therapy, may be helpful.
- **Monitor medications**: Some medications, such as antibiotics or corticosteroids, can disrupt the natural balance of bacteria and yeast in the body. Consulting with a healthcare professional about the potential impact of medications on Candida's growth is advisable.
- **Get enough sleep**: A lack of quality sleep can impair the immune system's ability to function optimally. Prioritizing adequate sleep can support overall immune health and help prevent Candida overgrowth.

These lifestyle changes can complement medical treatments prescribed by healthcare professionals. It's important to consult with a healthcare professional for an accurate diagnosis and appropriate treatment plan.

## Home Remedies for Candida Albicans

While medical treatments are the most effective way to address Candida Albicans infections, some individuals may also consider home remedies as complementary approaches. Here are some commonly suggested home remedies:

- **Coconut oil**: Raw organic coconut oil has antifungal properties and can be applied internally or externally to combat Candida Albicans yeast.
- **Yogurt and probiotics**: Consuming yogurt and probiotics rich in beneficial bacteria may help restore the natural balance of microorganisms in the body, potentially reducing Candida Albicans' overgrowth.
- **Garlic**: Garlic is known for its antimicrobial properties and may have an inhibitory effect on Candida Albicans. It can be consumed raw or added to meals.
- **Tea tree oil**: Tea tree oil has antifungal properties and can be diluted and applied topically to affected areas. However, caution should be exercised as it can cause skin irritation in some individuals.
- **Apple cider vinegar**: Apple cider vinegar is believed to have antifungal and antimicrobial effects. It may be used topically or added to bathwater for relief.
- **Boric acid**: Boric acid capsules or suppositories may be used in the vagina to help restore the pH balance and discourage the growth of Candida Albicans. However, it is important to use boric acid under the guidance of a healthcare professional.

These home remedies are often used in conjunction with medical treatments or as preventive measures. It is crucial to consult with a healthcare professional before trying any home remedies to ensure they are safe and appropriate for individual circumstances.

# Candida Albicans Diet

The Candida Albicans diet, also known as the Candida diet or anti-candida diet, is a dietary approach aimed at reducing the growth of Candida Albicans yeast in the body. This diet involves eliminating or minimizing foods that can promote yeast overgrowth, such as sugar, refined carbohydrates, yeast-containing foods, and certain dairy products.

The focus is on consuming nutrient-rich foods, including non-starchy vegetables, lean proteins, healthy fats, and probiotic-rich foods. The Candida Albicans diet aims to restore a healthy balance of microorganisms in the gut and support overall gut health. It is important to note that the Candida Albicans diet should be followed under the guidance of a healthcare professional or registered dietitian, as individual dietary needs may vary.

## Principles of the Candida Albicans Diet

The Candida Albicans diet is based on the following principles:

- **Eliminate added sugars**: The diet requires avoiding foods with added sugars, including processed sweets, sugary drinks, and high-sugar fruits.
- **Limit carbohydrates**: Carbohydrate intake is reduced to starve the yeast. This includes minimizing or eliminating refined carbohydrates like white bread, pasta, and pastries.
- **Avoid gluten**: Gluten-containing grains, such as wheat, barley, and rye, should be eliminated or limited due to their potential inflammatory effects.
- **Minimize alcohol consumption**: Alcoholic beverages, especially those high in sugar or yeast content, are best avoided during the Candida diet.
- **Exclude yeast-containing foods**: Foods that contain yeast or encourage yeast growth, such as bread, baked goods, fermented foods, and certain dairy products, should be minimized or eliminated.
- **Focus on nutrient-rich foods**: Non-starchy vegetables, lean proteins (such as poultry, fish, and plant-based sources), healthy fats (like avocados and olive oil), and probiotic-rich foods should form the foundation of the diet.
- **Support gut health**: The diet aims to promote a healthy balance of gut bacteria by consuming probiotic-rich foods and avoiding foods that can damage gut health.

Incorporating the principles of the Candida Albicans diet into everyday life can help reduce symptoms associated with yeast overgrowth and support overall health.

## Benefits of Candida Albicans Diet

This diet offers several potential benefits for individuals dealing with Candida overgrowth. Here are some benefits of following this diet:

- **Improved Digestive Health**: Following a candida albicans diet can lead to improved digestive health in women. By eliminating foods that promote Candida yeast growth, such as sugars and processed foods, the diet helps restore the balance of gut bacteria and reduce digestive issues like bloating and gas. This promotes better nutrient absorption and overall gut health.
- **Enhanced Energy Levels**: Women on a candida albicans diet often experience increased energy levels. By cutting out refined carbohydrates and sugars, the body relies on healthier sources of energy, such as lean proteins and complex carbohydrates. This helps stabilize blood sugar levels and prevents energy crashes, resulting in sustained energy throughout the day.
- **Strengthened Immune System**: The candida albicans diet can strengthen the immune system in women. By

eliminating inflammatory foods and promoting a nutrient-rich diet, the body is better equipped to fight off infections and diseases. This is especially beneficial for women prone to recurring yeast infections, as it helps reduce the growth of Candida fungi and promotes a healthier vaginal flora.

- **Weight Management**: Another benefit of the candida albicans diet for women is its potential for weight management. By avoiding foods that contribute to weight gain, such as refined sugars and processed carbohydrates, women may experience weight loss or maintain a healthy weight. Additionally, the diet's emphasis on whole, unprocessed foods can help curb cravings and promote a balanced approach to eating.

- **Improved Skin Health**: Following a candida albicans diet can lead to improved skin health in women. By reducing the consumption of inflammatory foods, such as sugar and processed foods, women may see a reduction in skin issues like acne and eczema. The diet's focus on nutrient-dense foods also provides essential vitamins and minerals that support skin health, promoting a clear and vibrant complexion.

In summary, the benefits of a candida albicans diet for women include improved digestive health, enhanced energy levels, a strengthened immune system, weight management, and improved skin health. By eliminating foods that promote Candida yeast growth and focusing on nutrient-rich options, women can experience these positive effects on their overall well-being.

## Disadvantages of Candida Albicans Diet

When following a Candida Albicans diet, there are some potential disadvantages to consider. However, the benefits of the diet generally outweigh these drawbacks. Here are five disadvantages of the Candida Albicans diet:

### Restrictive food choices

Avoiding sugar, gluten, alcohol, and caffeine can result in restrictive food choices on a candida albicans diet. While this approach is necessary to inhibit the growth of Candida yeast, it can make meal planning more challenging. Women following this diet may feel limited in their options and need to be creative to ensure a well-balanced and satisfying diet. However, with proper research and guidance, it is possible to find delicious alternatives and maintain a varied and nutritious eating plan.

### Nutrient deficiencies

Reducing or eliminating certain food groups as part of a Candida Albicans diet can hurt nutrient intake. This can be particularly problematic for carbohydrates, vitamins, and minerals. Carbohydrates are a vital energy source and play a key role in regulating blood sugar levels. Vitamins like vitamin C and B complex vitamins are essential for immune function and energy metabolism.

Similarly, minerals like calcium and iron are crucial for bone health and oxygen transport in the body. Careful meal planning is necessary to ensure adequate nutrient intake when following a Candida Albicans diet. It is recommended to consult a healthcare professional or registered dietitian to ensure a well-balanced and nutrient-rich diet.

**Social limitations**

Adhering to a Candida diet can have its drawbacks, particularly when it comes to socializing. It can be challenging to maintain dietary restrictions and avoid temptation when dining out or attending social gatherings. This can result in feelings of self-consciousness and exclusion, and possibly impact relationships and social experiences.

Additionally, the diet's limitations can make it difficult to find suitable options while traveling, further adding to the social limitations. While the diet's benefits are significant, it is essential to weigh the potential social repercussions before committing to it fully.

**Initial detox symptoms**

These initial detox symptoms can be a significant disadvantage for those starting the Candida diet. The sudden change in diet can cause the body to release toxins, leading to symptoms such as headaches, fatigue, and digestive discomfort. However, it is important to note that these symptoms are usually temporary and subside over time.

The body is adjusting to the new diet, and these symptoms are a sign that the body is getting rid of toxins. It is also important to remember that everyone's body is different, and the severity of these symptoms can vary.

Despite these potential disadvantages, the Candida Albicans diet offers several benefits. It can help reduce Candida overgrowth, alleviate symptoms such as bloating and fatigue, and promote overall gut health. As with any dietary change, it's recommended to consult with a healthcare professional or registered dietitian to ensure individual nutritional needs are met while following the Candida diet.

# 5 Step-Guide to Get Started with Candida Albicans Diet

Making significant dietary changes can seem challenging. Here is a step-by-step guide to help you get started with the Candida Albicans diet:

## Step 1: Consult a Healthcare Professional

It is essential to seek guidance from a healthcare professional before starting the Candida Albicans diet. Consulting with a healthcare professional allows for personalized advice tailored to your specific health needs and ensures that the diet is suitable for you. They will review your medical history, conduct any necessary tests, and provide expert guidance on how to safely and effectively proceed with the diet. Taking this precautionary step helps ensure that you embark on the Candida Albicans diet in a manner that supports your overall well-being.

## Step 2: Educate Yourself

While waiting for your consultation, take the initiative to educate yourself about Candida Albicans and the principles behind the diet. Research reputable sources, read books or articles written by experts in the field, and explore scientific studies related to Candida overgrowth. Understanding the condition and the diet will empower you to make informed decisions and actively participate in your journey toward better health.

## Step 3: Eliminate Sugar and High-Carb Foods

Following your healthcare professional's guidance, take action by eliminating sugar and high-carbohydrate foods from your diet. These foods contribute to yeast growth and can exacerbate Candida overgrowth. Remove items such as sugary snacks, sodas, pastries, and processed foods from your pantry. Instead, focus on consuming whole, unprocessed foods that are low in sugar and carbohydrates.

## Step 4: Remove Yeast-Containing Foods and Fermented Products

Continue implementing your healthcare professional's recommendations by removing yeast-containing foods and fermented products from your diet. These can fuel Candida's growth and hinder your progress. Avoid foods like bread, beer, wine, and certain cheeses that contain yeast. Be mindful of ingredients like vinegar, soy sauce, and pickles, which are commonly found in fermented products. Opt for fresh alternatives and flavorings instead.

## Step 5: Focus on Nutrient-Dense Foods

As you adhere to the dietary restrictions, prioritize nutrient-dense foods to support your overall health and immune system. Emphasize non-starchy vegetables like leafy greens, broccoli, cauliflower, and asparagus in your meals. Incorporate lean proteins such as chicken, fish, and tofu. Additionally, include healthy fats like avocados, olive oil, and nuts. These nutrient-rich choices will provide essential vitamins, minerals, and antioxidants for optimal well-being.

Throughout your Candida Albicans diet journey, maintain open communication with your healthcare professional. Regularly update them on your progress, share any challenges or concerns, and follow their guidance for monitoring and adjusting your dietary approach. With their support and your commitment, you can work towards rebalancing your gut health and managing Candida's overgrowth effectively.

## Foods to Eat

When following a Candida Albicans diet, it's important to choose foods that are low in sugar and carbohydrates and focus on nutrient-dense options. Here are some foods you can include in your diet:

- Non-Starchy Vegetables: Include plenty of non-starchy vegetables such as leafy greens (spinach, kale, lettuce), cruciferous vegetables (broccoli, cauliflower, Brussels sprouts), zucchini, cucumber, asparagus, and bell peppers.

- Lean Proteins: Opt for lean sources of protein like chicken, turkey, fish (salmon, trout, cod), eggs, tofu, tempeh, and legumes (lentils, chickpeas).
- Healthy Fats: Incorporate healthy fats into your meals, including avocados, olive oil, coconut oil, flaxseed oil, chia seeds, and nuts (almonds, walnuts, cashews).
- Low-Sugar Fruits: Choose fruits that are low in sugar, such as berries (blueberries, strawberries, raspberries), green apples, and citrus fruits (lemons, limes).
- Whole Grains: If tolerated, opt for gluten-free whole grains like quinoa, brown rice, buckwheat, and amaranth in moderation.
- Herbs and Spices: Flavor your dishes with herbs and spices that have antifungal properties, such as garlic, ginger, oregano, turmeric, cinnamon, and cayenne pepper.
- Beverages: Stay hydrated with water, herbal teas, and unsweetened almond or coconut milk. Avoid sugary drinks, fruit juices, and alcohol.

Remember to consult with a healthcare professional or registered dietitian for personalized guidance on your Candida Albicans diet. They can provide specific recommendations based on your individual needs and consider any other health conditions you may have.

# Foods To Avoid

When following a Candida Albicans diet, it's important to avoid certain foods that can promote yeast growth and worsen Candida overgrowth. Here are some foods to avoid:

- Sugar and Sweeteners: Avoid all forms of sugar, including white sugar, brown sugar, honey, maple syrup, and high-fructose corn syrup. Also, steer clear of artificial sweeteners like aspartame, sucralose, and saccharin.
- High-Carb Foods: Limit or eliminate high-carbohydrate foods that can break down into sugars in the body, such as white bread, pasta, rice, potatoes, and other refined grains.
- Yeast-Containing Foods: Avoid foods that contain yeast or are likely to promote yeast growth. This includes bread, buns, rolls, pastries, and other baked goods made with yeast.
- Fermented Products: Temporarily exclude fermented products like vinegar, soy sauce, pickles, and fermented vegetables, as they can contribute to yeast overgrowth.
- Alcohol: Alcoholic beverages should be avoided as they can disrupt the balance of gut bacteria and promote yeast growth. This includes beer, wine, liquor, and cocktails.

- Processed and Packaged Foods: Stay away from processed and packaged foods, as they often contain added sugars, preservatives, and other ingredients that can aggravate Candida's overgrowth.
- High-Sugar Fruits: While some low-sugar fruits can be enjoyed in moderation, it's best to avoid high-sugar fruits like bananas, grapes, mangoes, and dried fruits.
- Dairy Products: Dairy can be problematic for some individuals with Candida overgrowth. Avoid milk, cheese, yogurt, and other dairy products. Opt for non-dairy alternatives like almond milk or coconut milk.
- Caffeinated Beverages: It is best to limit or avoid caffeinated drinks like coffee and black tea, as they can disrupt the balance of beneficial bacteria in the gut.
- Processed Meats: Processed meats like sausages, deli meats, and hot dogs often contain preservatives and additives that can contribute to inflammation and weaken the immune system.

Remember, everyone's response to the Candida Albicans diet may vary. It's important to listen to your body, track your symptoms, and make adjustments as needed. Consult with a healthcare professional or registered dietitian for personalized guidance and recommendations tailored to your specific needs and health condition.

# Sample Recipes

Following a Candida Albicans diet doesn't have to be complicated. With proper planning and delicious recipes, you can easily manage your symptoms and heal your gut health. Here are some sample recipes to get you started.

# Baked Salmon with Lemon And Dili

**Ingredients:**

- Salmon filets
- Fresh lemon juice
- Fresh dill
- Salt
- Pepper

**Instructions:**

1. Preheat the oven to the recommended temperature for baking salmon (usually around 375°F or 190°C).

2. Place the salmon filets on a baking sheet lined with parchment paper or foil.

3. Squeeze fresh lemon juice over the salmon, ensuring each filet is coated. The amount of lemon juice can be adjusted based on personal preference.

4. Sprinkle fresh dill over the salmon filets, evenly distributing it among them.

5. Season with salt and pepper according to taste.

6. Carefully transfer the baking sheet to the preheated oven.

7. Bake the salmon for about 12-15 minutes, or until it is cooked through and flakes easily with a fork.

8. Once cooked, remove the salmon from the oven and let it rest for a few minutes before serving.

9. Serve the baked salmon hot, alongside your choice of side dishes or salad.

Note: Remember to adjust cooking times based on the thickness of the salmon filets to ensure they are fully cooked.

# Grilled Chicken Salad

## Ingredients:

- Chicken breast
- Mixed greens
- Cherry tomatoes
- Cucumbers
- Avocado
- Olive oil
- Lemon juice

## Instructions:

1. Grill the chicken breast until fully cooked.

2. Slice or shred the grilled chicken into bite-sized pieces.

3. In a large bowl, combine mixed greens, cherry tomatoes, sliced cucumbers, and diced avocado.

4. Add the grilled chicken to the salad.

5. Drizzle olive oil and lemon juice over the salad, tossing to coat everything evenly.

6. Season with salt and pepper to taste.

7. Serve the grilled chicken salad fresh and enjoy!

# Roasted Vegetable Medley

## Ingredients:

- Zucchini
- Bell peppers
- Broccoli
- Cauliflower
- Olive oil
- Garlic
- Herbs of choice (such as rosemary, thyme, or oregano)
- Salt
- Pepper

## Instructions:

1. Preheat your oven to a suitable roasting temperature, around 400°F (200°C).

2. Chop the zucchini, bell peppers, broccoli, and cauliflower into bite-sized pieces.

3. Place the chopped vegetables on a baking sheet lined with parchment paper.

4. Drizzle olive oil over the vegetables and sprinkle minced garlic, herbs, salt, and pepper.

5. Toss the vegetables to evenly coat them with the oil and seasonings.

6.  Spread the vegetables in a single layer on the baking sheet.

7.  Roast in the preheated oven for about 20-25 minutes or until the vegetables are tender and slightly caramelized.

8.  Remove from the oven and serve the roasted vegetables medley as a side dish or as a main course.

# Quinoa Stuffed Bell Peppers

## Ingredients:

- Bell peppers
- Quinoa
- Onion
- Garlic
- Spinach
- Diced tomatoes
- Olive oil
- Salt
- Pepper

## Instructions:

1. Preheat your oven to 375°F (190°C).

2. Cut the bell peppers in half lengthwise and remove the seeds and ribs.

3. Cook quinoa according to package instructions.

4. In a pan, sauté diced onion and minced garlic in olive oil until softened.

5. Add chopped spinach and cook until wilted.

6. Stir in cooked quinoa and diced tomatoes.

7. Season with salt and pepper to taste.

8. Fill each bell pepper half with the quinoa mixture.

9. Place the stuffed peppers in a baking dish.

10. Bake for about 20-25 minutes or until the peppers are soft and lightly browned.

11. Remove from the oven and serve the quinoa stuffed bell peppers as a nutritious and flavorful meal.

# Cauliflower Fried Rice

## Ingredients:

- Cauliflower florets
- Peas
- Carrots
- Onion
- Garlic
- Coconut aminos or soy sauce
- Olive oil
- Salt
- Pepper

## Instructions:

1. Process cauliflower florets in a food processor until they resemble rice grains.

2. In a large skillet or wok, heat olive oil over medium heat.

3. Add diced onion and minced garlic, and sauté until fragrant and translucent.

4. Add the riced cauliflower, peas, and shredded carrots to the skillet.

5. Stir-fry for about 5-7 minutes or until the cauliflower is tender and the vegetables are cooked.

6. Drizzle coconut aminos or soy sauce over the cauliflower mixture and toss to combine.

7. Season with salt and pepper to taste.

8. Continue to stir-fry for another 2-3 minutes until everything is well combined and heated through.

9. Remove from heat and serve the cauliflower fried rice as a low-carb alternative to traditional fried rice.

# Zucchini Noodles with Pesto

## Ingredients:

- Zucchini
- Fresh basil leaves
- Pine nuts
- Garlic
- Parmesan cheese (optional)
- Lemon juice
- Olive oil
- Cherry tomatoes

## Instructions:

1. Use a spiralizer or a julienne peeler to create zucchini noodles.

2. In a food processor, combine fresh basil leaves, pine nuts, minced garlic, and grated Parmesan cheese (optional).

3. Add a squeeze of lemon juice and drizzle olive oil into the food processor while blending until a smooth pesto sauce forms.

4. In a pan, sauté the zucchini noodles with a little olive oil until they are tender but still crisp.

5. Toss the zucchini noodles with the pesto sauce until evenly coated.

6. Top with halved cherry tomatoes and additional pine nuts for garnish, if desired.

7. Serve the zucchini noodles with pesto as a light and flavorful dish.

# Turkey Lettuce Wraps

**Ingredients:**

- Ground turkey
- Garlic
- Ginger
- Preferred seasonings (such as soy sauce, hoisin sauce, or chili paste)
- Lettuce leaves (such as butter lettuce or iceberg lettuce)
- Fresh cilantro
- Chopped peanuts (optional)

**Instructions:**

1. In a skillet, cook ground turkey over medium heat until browned.

2. Add minced garlic and grated ginger to the skillet and sauté for a minute until fragrant.

3. Stir in your preferred seasonings, such as soy sauce, hoisin sauce, or chili paste, to add flavor to the turkey.

4. Cook the turkey mixture for a few more minutes until it is fully cooked and well combined with the seasonings.

5. Wash and dry lettuce leaves, and separate them to create individual cups.

6. Spoon the cooked turkey mixture into each lettuce cup.

7. Garnish with fresh cilantro and chopped peanuts for added crunch and flavor.

8. Serve the turkey lettuce wraps as a light and satisfying meal or appetizer.

# Zucchini and Carrot Soup

## Ingredients:

- Zucchini
- Carrots
- Onion
- Garlic
- Vegetable broth
- Coconut milk (optional)
- Turmeric
- Cumin
- Salt
- Pepper

## Instructions:

1. Chop zucchini, carrots, onion, and garlic.

2. In a large pot, sauté the chopped vegetables in a little olive oil until they are slightly softened.

3. Add vegetable broth to the pot, enough to cover the vegetables.

4. Bring the mixture to a boil, then reduce heat and simmer until the vegetables are tender.

5. Use an immersion blender or transfer the mixture to a blender to puree until smooth.

6. Stir in coconut milk (if using), turmeric, cumin, salt, and pepper to taste.

7. Heat the soup again until warmed through.

8. Serve the zucchini and carrot soup as a comforting and nourishing meal.

# Quinoa and Vegetable Stir-Fry

## Ingredients:

- Quinoa
- Mixed vegetables (such as bell peppers, broccoli, and snap peas)
- Garlic
- Ginger
- Tamari sauce (gluten-free soy sauce)
- Sesame oil
- Coconut oil

## Instructions:

1. Cook quinoa according to package instructions.

2. In a large skillet or wok, heat coconut oil over medium heat.
   Add minced garlic and grated ginger to the skillet and sauté for a minute until fragrant.

3. Add mixed vegetables to the skillet and stir-fry until they are crisp-tender.

4. Drizzle tamari sauce and sesame oil over the vegetables, tossing to coat them evenly.

5. Add cooked quinoa to the skillet and stir-fry for another minute to combine all ingredients.

6. Season with salt and pepper if desired.

7. Serve the quinoa and vegetable stir-fry as a wholesome and flavorful dish.

# Cauliflower Pizza Crust

## Ingredients:

- Cauliflower florets
- Almond flour (or other gluten-free flour)
- Nutritional yeast (optional)
- Garlic powder (optional)
- Onion powder (optional)
- Salt
- Eggs
- Olive oil

## Instructions:

1. Preheat the oven to 400°F.

2. Pulse cauliflower florets in a food processor until they resemble rice grains.

3. Spread the cauliflower on a baking sheet lined with parchment paper and bake for about 15-20 minutes or until lightly golden brown. Allow to cool slightly before transferring it to a bowl.

4. Add almond flour, nutritional yeast (optional), garlic and onion powder (optional), and salt to the bowl with cooled cauliflower, stirring to combine.

5. Whisk eggs in a separate bowl, then pour over the cauliflower mixture.

6. Stir until everything is well combined and the dough starts to form.

7. Drizzle olive oil on top of the dough and knead it into the dough until it forms into a ball.

8. Place the dough onto a parchment paper-lined baking sheet and shape it into a pizza crust.

9. Bake the cauliflower pizza crust in a preheated oven for about 30 minutes or until golden brown on top and bottom.

10. Once done, remove from the oven and let cool before adding desired toppings.

11. Bake the pizza for an additional 10 minutes or until the toppings are cooked through and melted (if using cheese).

12. Serve the cauliflower pizza crust as a delicious and healthier alternative to traditional pizza.

# Cucumber and Avocado Sushi Rolls

## Ingredients:

- Nori seaweed sheets
- Cooked quinoa
- Cucumber, julienned
- Avocado, sliced
- Tamari sauce (gluten-free soy sauce)
- Wasabi paste (optional)
- Pickled ginger (optional)

## Instructions:

1. Place a nori seaweed sheet on a sushi mat or a clean kitchen towel.

2. Spread a thin layer of cooked quinoa evenly over the nori sheet, leaving a small border at the top.

3. Arrange cucumber and avocado slices on top of the quinoa.

4. Drizzle tamari sauce over the filling ingredients.

5. Starting from the bottom, tightly roll the sushi using the mat or towel to help keep it compact.

6. Moisten the top border with a little water to seal the roll.

7. Use a sharp knife to slice the sushi roll into bite-sized pieces.

8. Serve the cucumber and avocado sushi rolls with tamari sauce, wasabi paste (if desired), and pickled ginger for a delicious and refreshing snack or light meal.

# Creamy Coconut Yogurt Bowl with Crunchy Granola and Sweet Berries

## Ingredients:

- 1 cup of unsweetened coconut yogurt
- 1/4 cup of your favorite granola
- A handful of fresh mixed berries (such as strawberries, blueberries, and raspberries)
- Optional toppings: drizzle of honey or maple syrup, shredded coconut, or chopped nuts

## Instructions:

1. Start by spooning a generous portion of unsweetened coconut yogurt into a serving bowl.

2. Sprinkle the creamy coconut yogurt with a quarter cup of your favorite granola, distributing it evenly across the surface.

3. Top the granola with a vibrant mix of fresh berries, using a handful to add color and natural sweetness to the bowl.

4. For added flavor and texture, feel free to drizzle a small amount of honey or maple syrup over the berries.

5. If desired, garnish the coconut yogurt bowl with a sprinkle of shredded coconut or a handful of chopped nuts for an extra crunch.

6. Serve immediately and enjoy this delightful combination of creamy coconut yogurt, crunchy granola, and sweet berries!

Feel free to adjust the quantities of each ingredient based on your preferences. You can also get creative by adding additional toppings such as chia seeds or sliced bananas.

# Poached Eggs with Spinach and Mushrooms

## Ingredients:

- 2 fresh eggs
- 2 cups fresh spinach leaves, washed and dried
- 1 cup sliced mushrooms (any variety)
- 1 tablespoon olive oil
- Salt and pepper to taste
- Optional toppings: grated Parmesan cheese, chopped fresh herbs (such as parsley or chives)

## Instructions:

1. Fill a medium-sized saucepan with water, about halfway full, and bring it to a gentle simmer over medium heat.

2. While the water is heating up, heat olive oil in a large non-stick skillet over medium heat.

3. Add the sliced mushrooms to the skillet and sauté until they become tender and lightly golden brown. This process should take about 5-6 minutes. Season them with salt and pepper to taste.

4. Once the mushrooms are cooked, add the fresh spinach leaves to the skillet. Stir occasionally until the spinach wilts down, approximately 2-3 minutes. Season with a pinch of salt and pepper if desired.

5. Once the water in the saucepan is gently simmering, carefully crack one egg into a small bowl or ramekin, making sure not to break the yolk. Slowly slide the egg into the simmering water, trying to keep it intact. Repeat this process with the second egg.

6. Allow the eggs to poach undisturbed for about 3-4 minutes until the whites are set, but the yolks are still slightly runny. Adjust the cooking time based on your preference for the runniness or firmness of the yolks.

7. Use a slotted spoon to carefully remove the poached eggs from the water, allowing any excess water to drain off.

8. Divide the sautéed spinach and mushrooms equally into two serving plates. Gently place one poached egg on top of each pile of spinach and mushrooms.

9. Sprinkle with grated Parmesan cheese and chopped fresh herbs if desired.

10. Serve the poached eggs with sautéed spinach and mushrooms immediately, allowing the runny yolks to mingle with the flavors of the vegetables for a delicious and nourishing meal.

# Salmon Salad with Avocado Dressing

## Ingredients:

- 1 salmon filet
- 4 cups mixed salad greens
- 1 cucumber, sliced
- 1 avocado, peeled, pitted, and diced
- 1/4 cup chopped red onion
- 1/4 cup cherry tomatoes, halved
- Freshly squeezed juice of 1 lemon
- Salt and pepper to taste

For the Avocado Dressing:

- 1 ripe avocado
- 1/4 cup plain Greek yogurt
- 2 tablespoons fresh cilantro, chopped
- 1 tablespoon lime juice
- 1 clove garlic, minced
- Salt and pepper to taste
- Water (if needed to thin out the dressing)

## Instructions:

1. Preheat your oven to 400°F (200°C). Season the salmon filet with salt and pepper, and place it on a baking sheet lined with parchment paper. Bake for about 12-15 minutes or until the salmon is cooked

through and flakes easily with a fork. Set aside to cool slightly.

2.  In a large salad bowl, combine the mixed salad greens, sliced cucumber, diced avocado, chopped red onion, and cherry tomatoes.

3.  In a small bowl, prepare the avocado dressing by mashing the ripe avocado with a fork until smooth. Add the Greek yogurt, fresh cilantro, lime juice, minced garlic, salt, and pepper. Stir well to combine. If the dressing is too thick, you can add a little water to thin it out to your desired consistency.

4.  Drizzle the avocado dressing over the salad ingredients and gently toss until everything is well coated.

5.  Flake the baked salmon into bite-sized pieces and arrange it on top of the salad.

6.  Squeeze fresh lemon juice over the salad for an extra burst of flavor. Season with additional salt and pepper to taste.

7.  Serve the Salmon Salad with Avocado Dressing immediately, enjoying the creamy and refreshing combination of flavors.

Feel free to customize your salad by adding other vegetables or toppings of your choice. This recipe is a delicious and healthy way to enjoy the goodness of salmon combined with the creaminess of avocado dressing.

# 7-Day Meal Plan

Planning ahead of time can make it easier to stick to a candida albicans diet. With a few tasty and nourishing meals, it is possible to manage this condition healthily. Below is a sample meal plan for a week, for breakfast, lunch, dinner, and snack time. Take note that you can change the order of the meals or even change the meals with appropriate choices according to your preference.

## Day 1

Breakfast

- Quinoa Porridge with Fruit

Lunch

- Turkey Lettuce Wraps

Dinner

- Zucchini and Carrot Soup

Snack

- Apple slices with almond butter

## Day 2

Breakfast

- Poached Eggs with Spinach and Mushrooms

Lunch

- Salmon Salad with Avocado Dressing

Dinner

- Quinoa and Vegetable Stir-Fry

Snack

- Hummus with carrot sticks or celery

## **Day 3**

Breakfast

- Scrambled Eggs with Tomatoes

Lunch

- Cauliflower Tacos

Dinner

- Baked Salmon with Roasted Asparagus

Snack

- Celery sticks with nut butter

## **Day 4**

Breakfast

- Sweet Potato Toast with Avocado and Egg

Lunch

- Chickpea Salad Sandwich

Dinner

- Stuffed Bell Peppers

Snack

- Apple slices with nut butter

## Day 5

Breakfast

- Coconut Yogurt with Granola and Berries

Lunch

- Salmon Burgers with Avocado Salad

Dinner

- Zucchini Noodles with Turkey Meatballs

Snack

- Celery sticks with hummus

## Day 6

Breakfast

- Egg Scramble with Spinach and Mushrooms

Lunch

- Turkey Lettuce Wraps

Dinner

- Baked Salmon with Roasted Asparagus

Snack

- Apple slices with nut butter

**Day 7**

Breakfast

- Coconut Yogurt with Granola and Berries

Lunch

- Cauliflower Pizza Crust

Dinner

- Quinoa and Vegetable Stir-Fry

Snack

- Hummus with carrot sticks or celery

Following a meal plan like this is beneficial for you as it helps not only stick to your diet but also manage your time in prepping your food. Consult with your doctor or a dietitian regarding the meal plan you want to follow, so medical professionals can help you curate the diet to better cater to your needs.

# Conclusion

Congratulations! You've reached the end of this comprehensive guide on Candida Albicans and the power of a Candida Albicans Diet. By making it this far, you've taken an important step towards regaining control over your health and well-being. We understand that dealing with Candida Albicans, especially in women, can be challenging and frustrating. But don't worry, you're not alone in this journey.

Throughout this guide, we've explored the ins and outs of Candida Albicans, its symptoms, causes, and the impact it can have on your life. We've delved into the importance of diet and how it can play a pivotal role in managing this condition. By adopting a Candida Albicans Diet, you're taking a proactive approach to restoring balance in your body and reclaiming your vitality.

One of the key insights we've discovered is that Candida Albicans thrives on sugar. By reducing your sugar intake, you're effectively starving the yeast and hindering its ability to grow and spread. The Candida Albicans Diet focuses on eliminating refined sugars, processed foods, and alcohol while emphasizing nutrient-dense, whole foods. This approach not only helps to rebalance your gut flora but also strengthens your immune system.

Another important aspect we covered is the significance of probiotics. Probiotics are beneficial bacteria that help restore the natural balance of your gut microbiome. Incorporating probiotic-rich foods like yogurt, sauerkraut, and kefir into your Candida Albicans Diet can provide your body with the essential support it needs to fight off the overgrowth of Candida.

Additionally, we emphasized the importance of stress management and self-care. Stress can weaken your immune system and disrupt the delicate balance in your body, making you more susceptible to Candida Albicans. By incorporating relaxation techniques, exercise, and mindfulness practices into your daily routine, you're creating a supportive environment for your body to heal and thrive.

Remember, managing Candida Albicans is a journey, and it may take time to see significant improvements. Be patient with yourself and celebrate each small victory along the way. Keep in mind that everyone's body is unique, and what works for one person may not work for another. It's essential to listen to your body and make adjustments to your Candida Albicans Diet as needed.

While adopting a Candida Albicans Diet is a crucial step, it's equally important to seek guidance from a healthcare professional. They can provide personalized recommendations and monitor your progress throughout your Candida Albicans journey. Remember, you don't have to face this alone – there are countless resources available to support you on your path to wellness.

As you wrap up this guide, we encourage you to stay positive and motivated. You have already taken the first step towards overcoming Candida Albicans by educating yourself and committing to a Candida Albicans Diet. Trust in the process and believe in your ability to regain control of your health.

We hope this guide has empowered you with the knowledge and tools you need to embark on your journey to better health. Remember, healing takes time, but with patience and perseverance, you can conquer Candida Albicans and live a vibrant, fulfilling life.

# FAQs

**What is Candida Albicans, and how does it affect women?**

Candida Albicans is a type of yeast that naturally exists in the body, including the vaginal area. However, when its growth becomes uncontrolled, it can lead to various health issues, particularly in women. Symptoms may include vaginal yeast infections, itching, burning, and discharge.

**What causes an overgrowth of Candida Albicans in women?**

Several factors can contribute to the overgrowth of Candida Albicans in women. These include a weakened immune system, hormonal changes (such as during pregnancy or menopause), taking antibiotics, high sugar intake, stress, and wearing tight-fitting or damp clothing.

**What is a Candida Albicans Diet, and how does it help manage the condition?**

A Candida Albicans Diet involves eliminating foods that promote yeast growth, such as refined sugars, processed foods, alcohol, and certain carbohydrates. Instead, the diet emphasizes whole foods, low-sugar fruits, non-starchy vegetables, lean proteins, healthy fats, and probiotic-rich foods. This helps restore balance in the gut and reduce Candida overgrowth.

## Can a Candida Albicans Diet help with other symptoms besides yeast infections?

Yes, adopting a Candida Albicans Diet may have positive effects on other symptoms associated with Candida overgrowth. These can include fatigue, brain fog, digestive issues, skin problems, and recurrent urinary tract infections. By addressing the root cause, the diet aims to alleviate these symptoms and improve overall well-being.

## How long does it take to see results from a Candida Albicans Diet?

The time it takes to see results from a Candida Albicans Diet varies from person to person. Some individuals may experience improvements within weeks, while others may take longer. It's important to be patient and consistent with the diet, as it can take time for the body to rebalance and for symptoms to subside.

## Can I follow a Candida Albicans Diet while taking medications?

It's crucial to consult with a healthcare professional before starting any diet, especially if you're on medication. They can guide how to integrate the Candida Albicans Diet with your current treatment plan. In some cases, modifications may be necessary to ensure optimal health and safety.

**Are there any additional lifestyle changes that can support a Candida Albicans Diet?**

In addition to dietary changes, certain lifestyle adjustments can complement a Candida Albicans Diet. These include managing stress levels, getting enough sleep, practicing good hygiene, avoiding tight-fitting or damp clothing, and incorporating regular exercise. These changes can help support the body's natural defenses and promote overall wellness.

Remember, it's essential to work closely with a healthcare professional when dealing with Candida Albicans. They can provide personalized advice and monitor your progress to ensure the most effective management of your condition.

# Resources and Helpful Links

Kumwenda, P., Cottier, F., Hendry, A. C., Kneafsey, D., Keevan, B., Gallagher, H., Tsai, H., & Hall, R. (2022). Estrogen promotes the innate immune evasion of Candida albicans through inactivation of the alternative complement system. Cell Reports, 38(1), 110183. https://doi.org/10.1016/j.celrep.2021.110183

Professional, C. C. M. (n.d.). Candida albicans. Cleveland Clinic. https://my.clevelandclinic.org/health/diseases/22961-candida-albicans#:~:text=Is%20Candida%20albicans%20an%20infection,overgrowth%20of%20yeast%20(Candida).

Mitchell Medical Group. (2023, July 22). Top 10 Candida overgrowth symptoms | Top NYC Candida Doctor. https://www.mitchellmedicalgroup.com/services/candida/top-10-candida-symptoms/

Richards, L. (2021, December 14). Foods To Eat On The Candida Diet. The Candida Diet. https://www.thecandidadiet.com/foodstoeat.htm

Richards, L. (2021a, January 15). 6 Benefits of the Candida Diet » The Candida Diet. The Candida Diet. https://www.thecandidadiet.com/benefits-of-the-candida-diet/

Richards, L. (2021c, December 14). Foods To Eat On The Candida Diet. The Candida Diet.

https://www.thecandidadiet.com/foodstoeat.htm#:~:text=Look%20for%2
0foods%20that%20are,fermented%20foods%20and%20bone%20broth.

Expert, Y. I. C. (2021, December 31). 5 Foods To Avoid In Candida Diet Yeast Infection [& List of Foods To Eat] | Medium. Medium. https://medium.com/@yeast-infection-cure/foods-to-avoid-in-candida-di et-577d4fc07689

9 798869 285515